I Can Cope!

I USE YOGA TO COPE

CAITIE MCANENEY

PowerKiDS press

Published in 2023 by The Rosen Publishing Group, Inc.
2544 Clinton Street, Buffalo, NY 14224

First Edition

Book Design: Michael Flynn

Photo Credits: Cover Galovtsik Gabor/Shutterstock.com; (series background) Abscent Vector/Shutterstock.com; pp. 5, 18 wavebreakmedia/Shutterstock.com; p. 7 Bondar Illia/Shutterstock.com; p. 8 vectorfusionart/Shutterstock.com; p. 9 Prostock-studio/Shutterstock.com; pp. 11 (all), 13 (top) narikan/Shutterstock.com; p. 13 (bottom) Kat Om/Shutterstock.com; p. 15 (main) Vasyl Nagernyak/Shutterstock.com; p. 15 (inset) n.k. junky/Shutterstock.com; p. 17 Pixel-Shot/Shutterstock.com; p. 19 Olesya Turchuk/Shutterstock.com; p. 21 Roman Samborskyi/Shutterstock.com.

Library of Congress Cataloging-in-Publication Data

Names: McAneney, Caitie, author.
Title: I use yoga to cope / Caitie McAneney.
Description: Buffalo, New York : PowerKids Press, [2023] | Series: I can cope! | Includes bibliographical references and index.
Identifiers: LCCN 2022028026 (print) | LCCN 2022028027 (ebook) | ISBN 9781538389577 (library binding) | ISBN 9781538389553 (paperback) | ISBN 9781538389584 (ebook)
Subjects: LCSH: Yoga–Juvenile literature. | Hatha yoga for children–Juvenile literature. | Mind and body in children–Juvenile literature.
Classification: LCC RJ133.7 .M33 2023 (print) | LCC RJ133.7 (ebook) | DDC 613.7/046083–dc23/eng/20220713
LC record available at https://lccn.loc.gov/2022028026
LC ebook record available at https://lccn.loc.gov/2022028027

Manufactured in the United States of America

Some of the images in this book illustrate individuals who are models. The depictions do not imply actual situations or events.

CPSIA Compliance Information: Batch #CWPK23. For Further Information contact Rosen Publishing at 1-800-237-9932.

CONTENTS

Cope and Connect

Have you ever felt so **anxious** that your belly hurt? Or so angry that your jaw or fists felt tense, or tight? Bodies and minds are connected, or joined. When you have big feelings like anger, sadness, or anxiety, you can feel them in your body. Luckily, you can also use the mind-body connection to **cope**.

The word "yoga" means "to join" or "to unite." The practice of yoga creates **harmony** between the mind and body. It helps people find a sense of peace.

COPING TOOLBOX

YOGA IS A PRACTICE FROM **ANCIENT** INDIA. YOGA TERMS ARE OFTEN IN **SANSKRIT**.

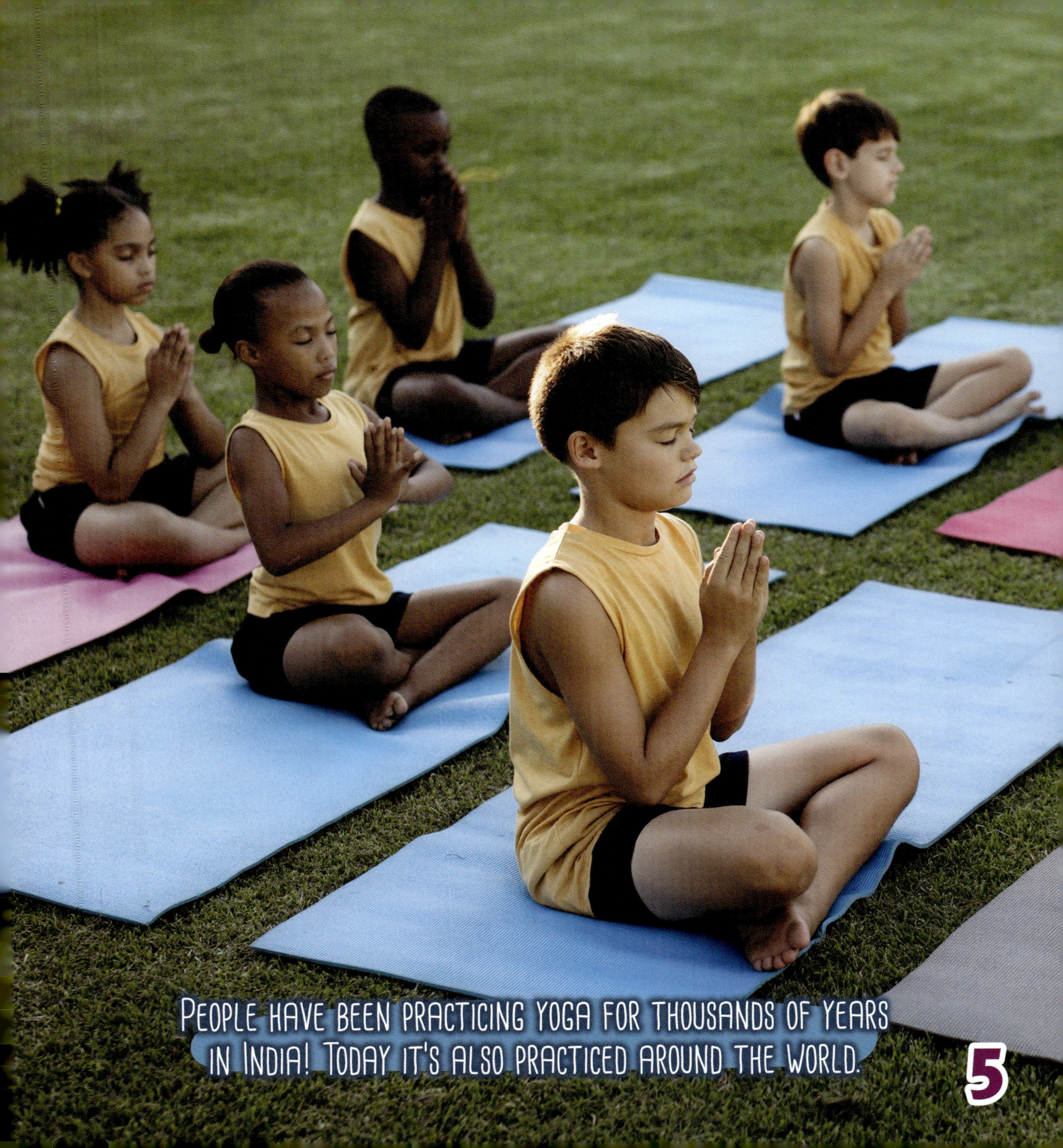

PEOPLE HAVE BEEN PRACTICING YOGA FOR THOUSANDS OF YEARS IN INDIA! TODAY IT'S ALSO PRACTICED AROUND THE WORLD.

What Is Yoga?

Yoga isn't just about bending into twisty **poses**. People of any age, ability, body size, or background can practice yoga. Everything you need is within you.

This ancient practice has eight limbs, or parts. The first two limbs include teachings about how to live, such as treating all beings with **nonviolence**. The next limb, *asana* (AH-suh-nuh), includes yoga poses. The other limbs cover breathing, **focus**, and **meditating**. Many believe practicing the eight limbs of yoga leads to great peace and well-being.

COPING TOOLBOX

YOGA HELPS PEOPLE RELAX, OR CALM, THEIR BODY AND MIND. THIS HELPS PEOPLE DEAL WITH NEGATIVE ENERGY, OR STRESS.

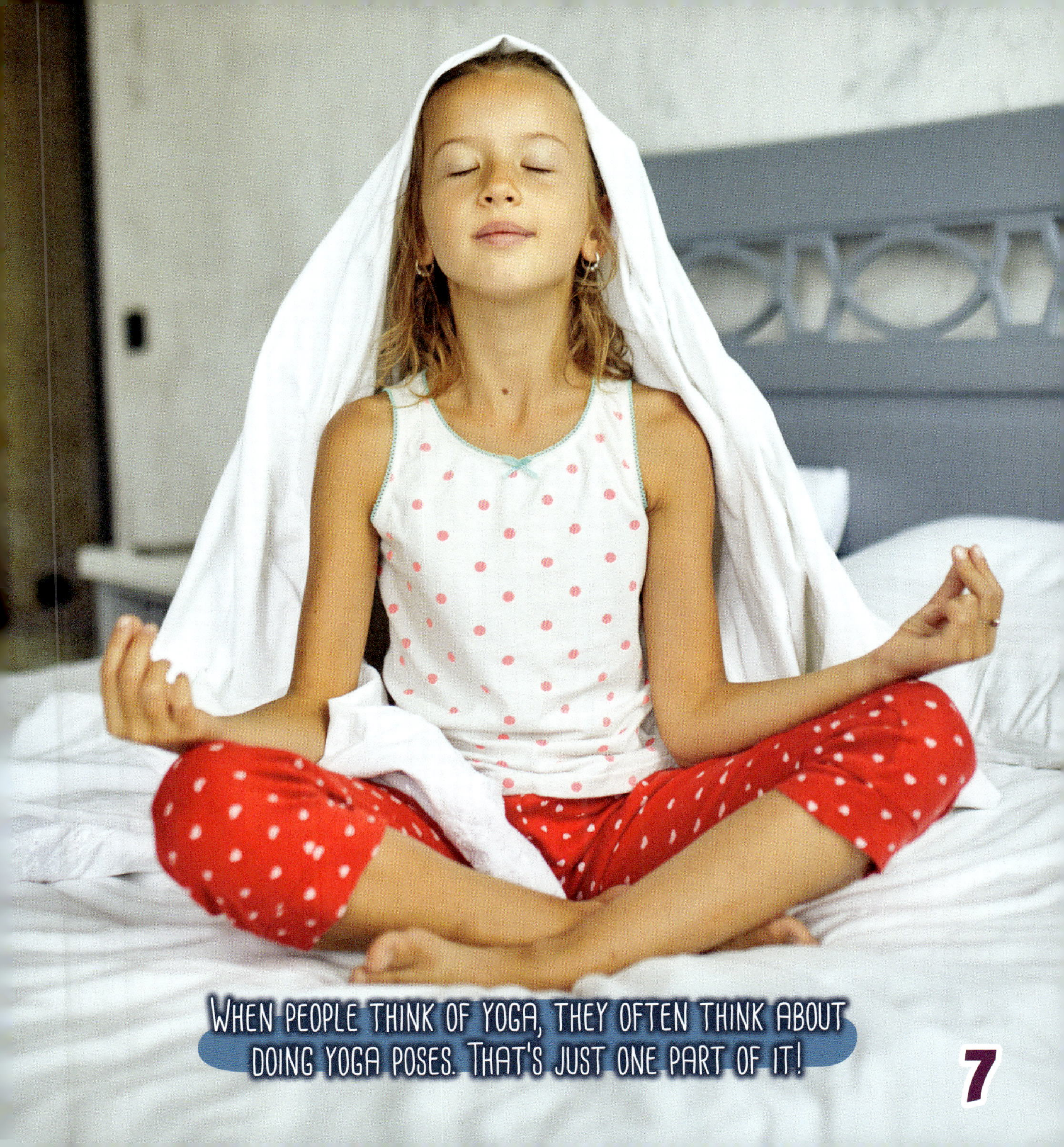

WHEN PEOPLE THINK OF YOGA, THEY OFTEN THINK ABOUT DOING YOGA POSES. THAT'S JUST ONE PART OF IT!

Getting Started

If you can, find a quiet place to do yoga. A mat is helpful but not always needed if you don't have one.

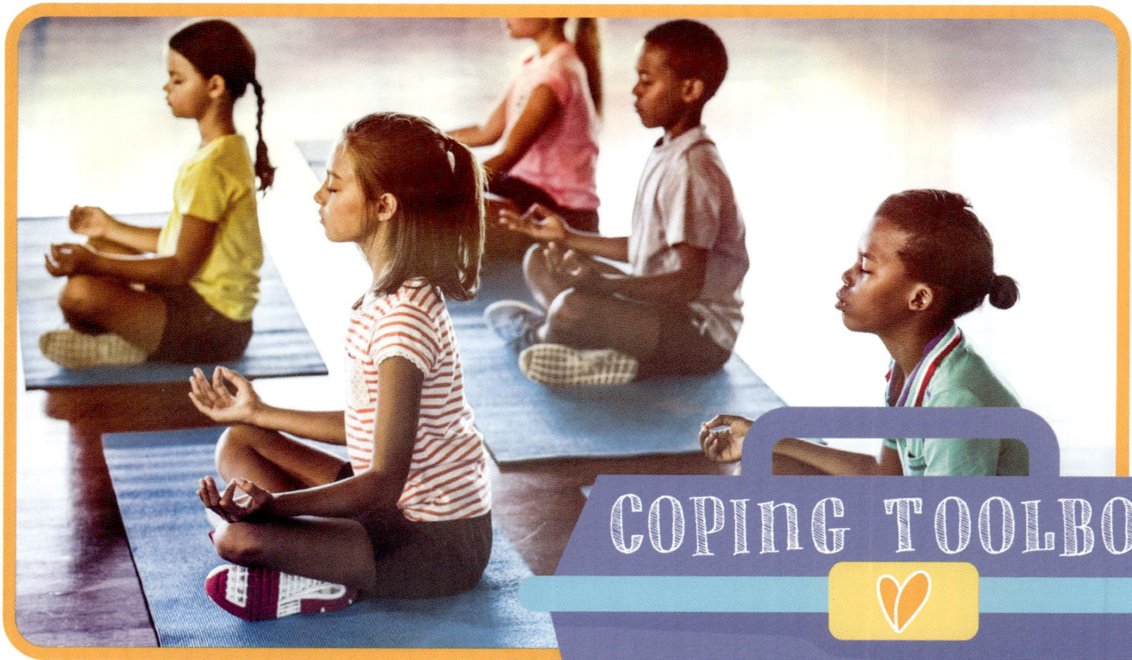

COPING TOOLBOX

IN YOGA, SITTING WITH YOUR LEGS CROSSED IS OFTEN CALLED "EASY POSE" OR "COMFORT POSE." YOU CAN SIT UP ON A PILLOW FOR MORE COMFORT.

To begin, find a comfortable seat on the ground. Close your eyes. Feel the way the ground supports, or holds, your body. Put your hands on your knees, palms up or down. Or, you can put one hand on your heart and one hand on your belly. Just breathe here. Become mindful, or aware, of what's going on inside you. As your body settles, your mind will too.

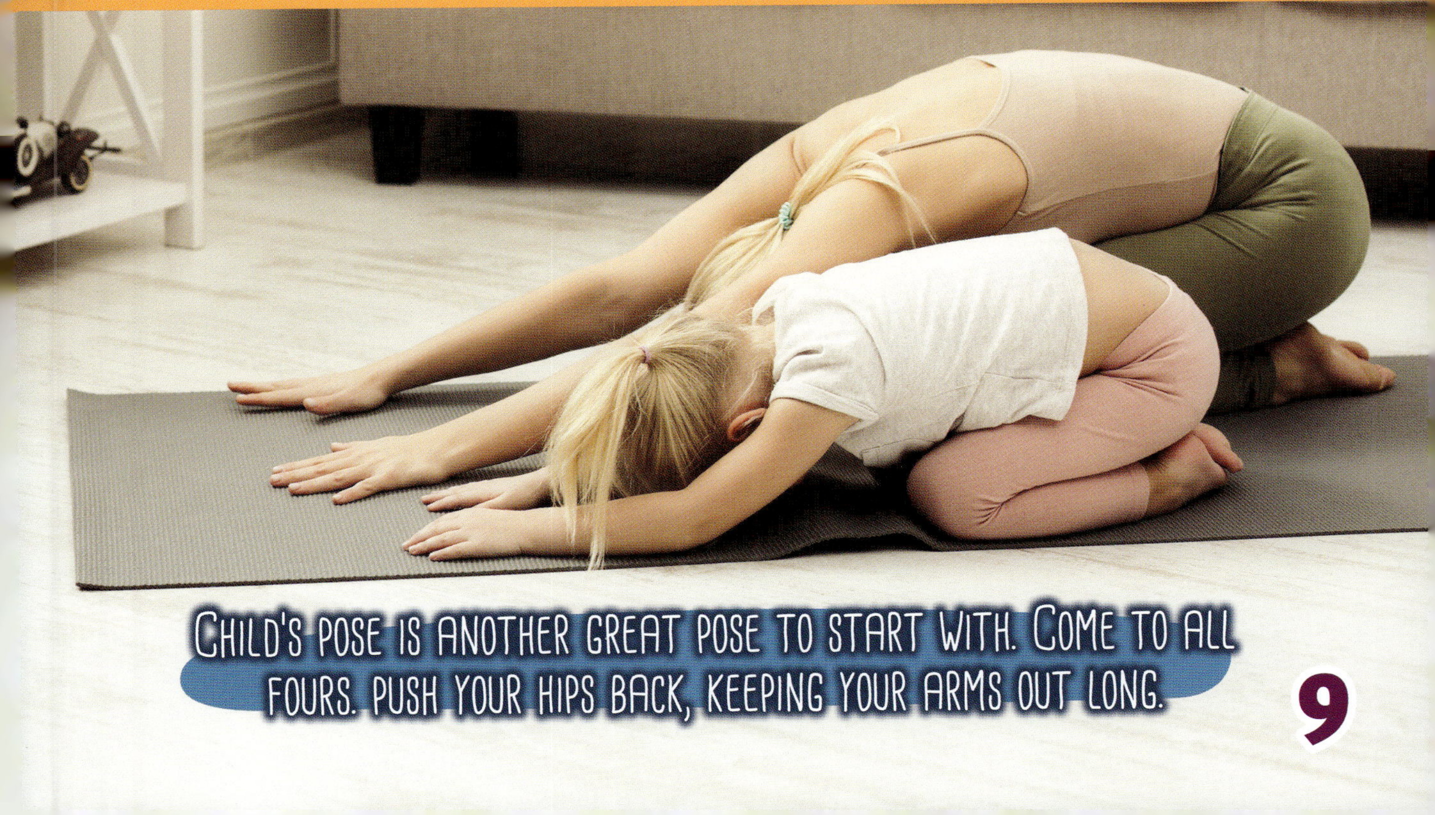

CHILD'S POSE IS ANOTHER GREAT POSE TO START WITH. COME TO ALL FOURS. PUSH YOUR HIPS BACK, KEEPING YOUR ARMS OUT LONG.

Warm-Up Movements

It's important to warm up your **muscles**. As you sit, bring your fingertips to the ground on either side of you. Then, on your inhale (in breath), sweep your hands overhead until your fingertips touch. On your exhale (out breath) bring them back to the ground. Do this for a few rounds of breath.

For a side body stretch, reach up and join your hands. Bend to one side, then the other. Then, move your shoulders, neck, and wrists around in any way that feels good!

COPING TOOLBOX

CAT AND COW ARE GREAT WARM-UP POSES. COME TO ALL FOURS. ROUND YOUR BACK LIKE A CAT. THEN, DROP YOUR BELLY LIKE A COW.

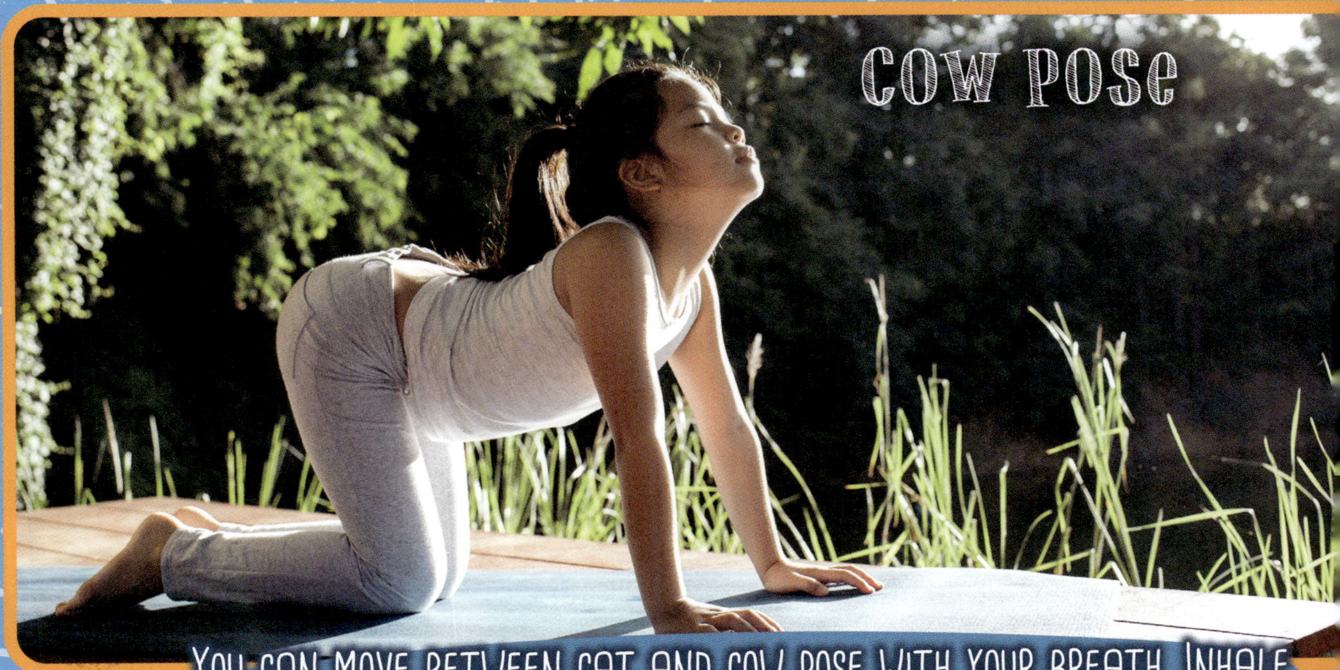

YOU CAN MOVE BETWEEN CAT AND COW POSE WITH YOUR BREATH. INHALE INTO COW, EXHALE INTO CAT. REPEAT IT FOR FIVE ROUNDS OF BREATH.

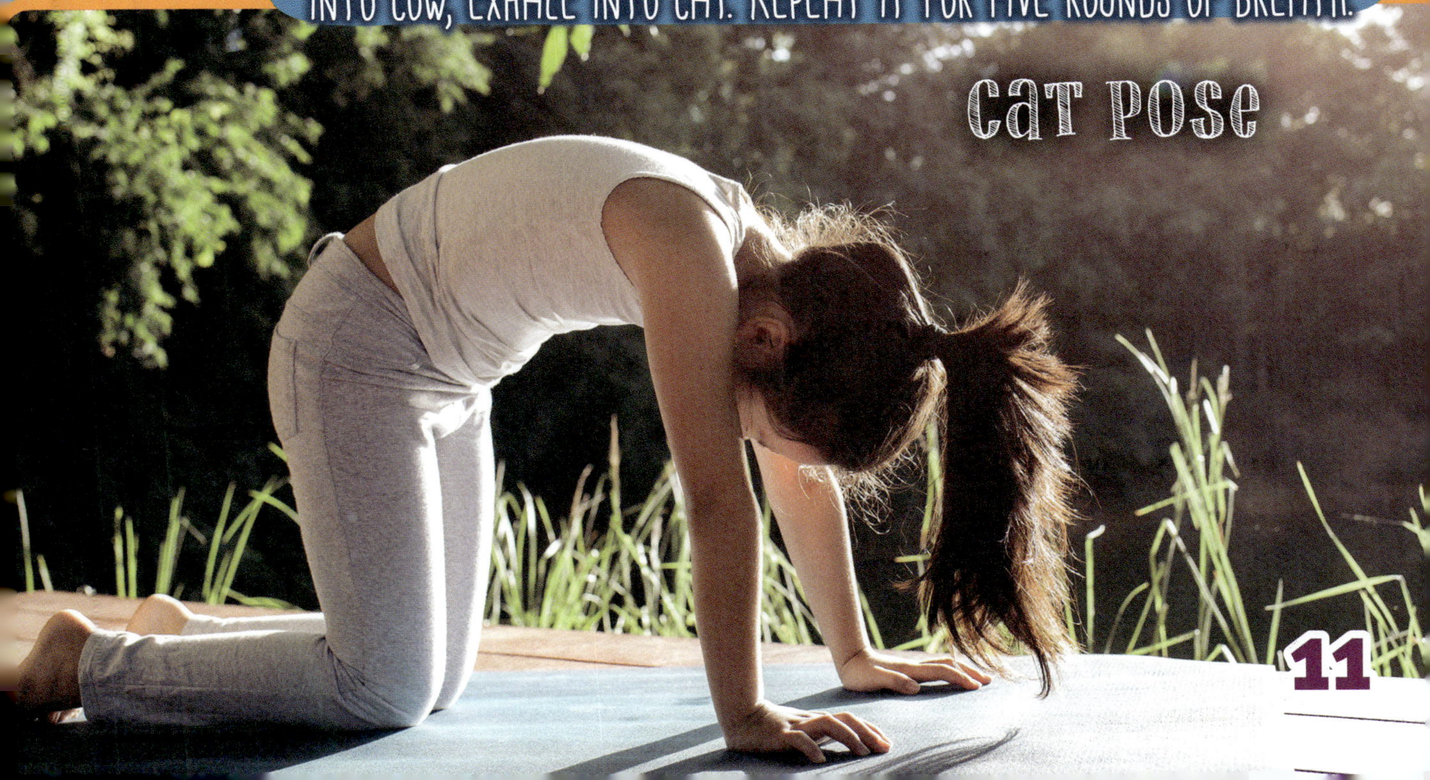

Move with Breath

Moving your body to your breath helps you further connect to your body. One special set of poses is called a sun salutation. You do each move with an inhale or exhale.

For a half sun salutation, stand in mountain pose. Inhale, reach up high. Exhale, bend forward to touch your toes. Inhale, put your hands on your thighs, look forward, and lift halfway so your back is flat. Exhale, bend again. Inhale, stretch your arms up high. Exhale, bring your hands together at your heart.

COPING TOOLBOX

IN MOUNTAIN POSE, STAND UP TALL. IMAGINE YOU HAVE ROOTS CONNECTING YOUR FEET TO THE GROUND AND A STRING CONNECTING YOUR HEAD TO THE SKY.

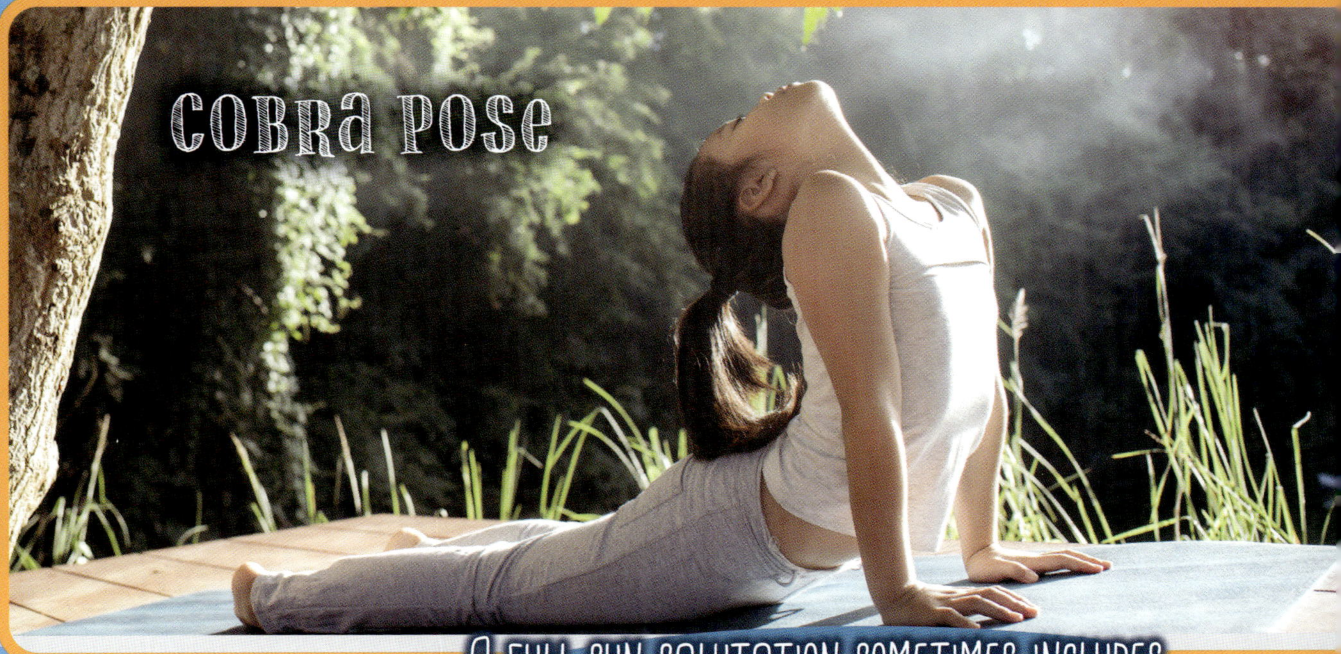

Cobra Pose

A FULL SUN SALUTATION SOMETIMES INCLUDES COBRA POSE AND DOWNWARD FACING DOG POSE.

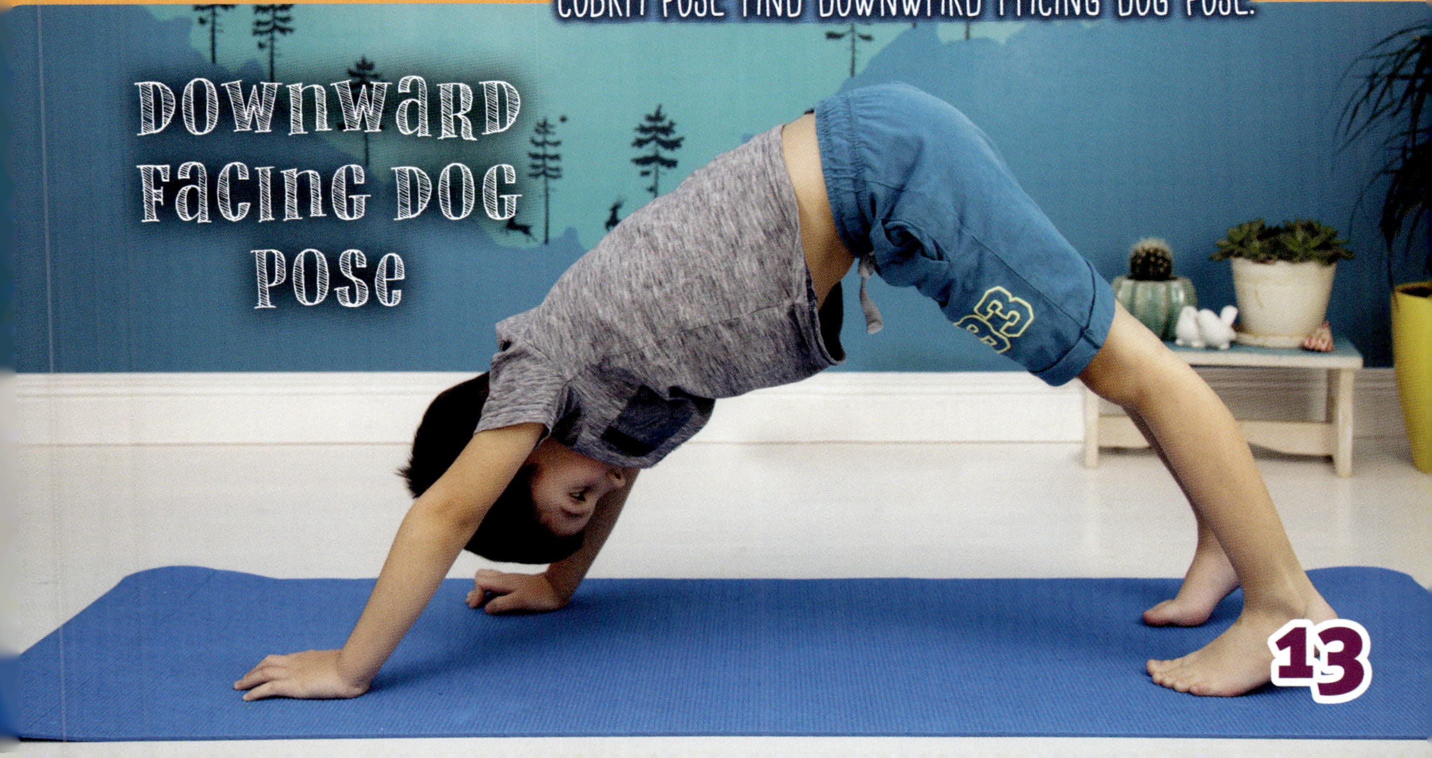

Downward Facing Dog Pose

Stand Strong

Standing poses help you build strength. Your leg muscles may feel some heat!

There are five warrior poses. For Warrior 2 pose, stand with your legs wide. Point your right toes to the short side and left toes to the long side of your mat. Bend your right knee. Bring your arms up in line with the floor. Look past your right middle finger. Feel power in your core (near your belly). Imagine pressing down with this power through your feet. Switch sides. You are a strong warrior!

COPING TOOLBOX

STANDING POSES CAN MAKE YOU FEEL POWERFUL. THIS MIGHT HELP WHEN YOU FEEL SAD, WORRIED, OR DOWN.

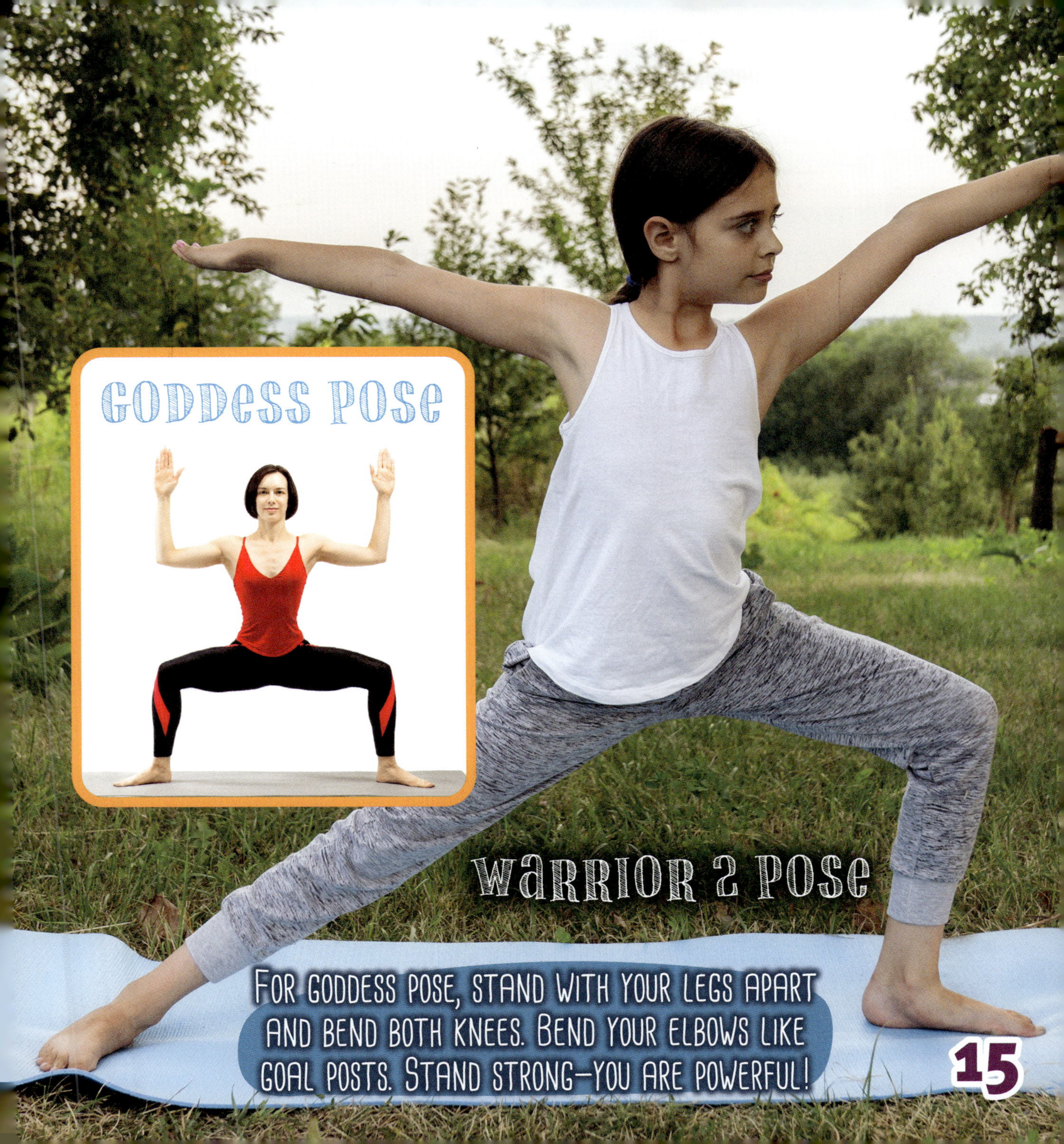

Goddess Pose

Warrior 2 Pose

For goddess pose, stand with your legs apart and bend both knees. Bend your elbows like goal posts. Stand strong—you are powerful!

Find Your Balance

It can be really hard to **balance**, especially when you're upset. Balancing poses help you focus. That helps you deal with stress.

Tree pose is a challenging standing pose. First, stand tall in mountain pose. Lift up your left foot. Place it either on your right ankle, shin, or thigh. Feel the wiggle in your body and work to find your balance. Then, raise your hands over your head. You can also bring your hands together at your heart. Try it on both sides!

COPING TOOLBOX

TO FIND BALANCE IN A HARD POSE, IT'S HELPFUL TO FOCUS ON A SPOT IN FRONT OF YOU. IT CAN BE A PICTURE, A LEAF, OR A CRACK IN A WALL. THIS FOCUS WILL KEEP YOU STEADY.

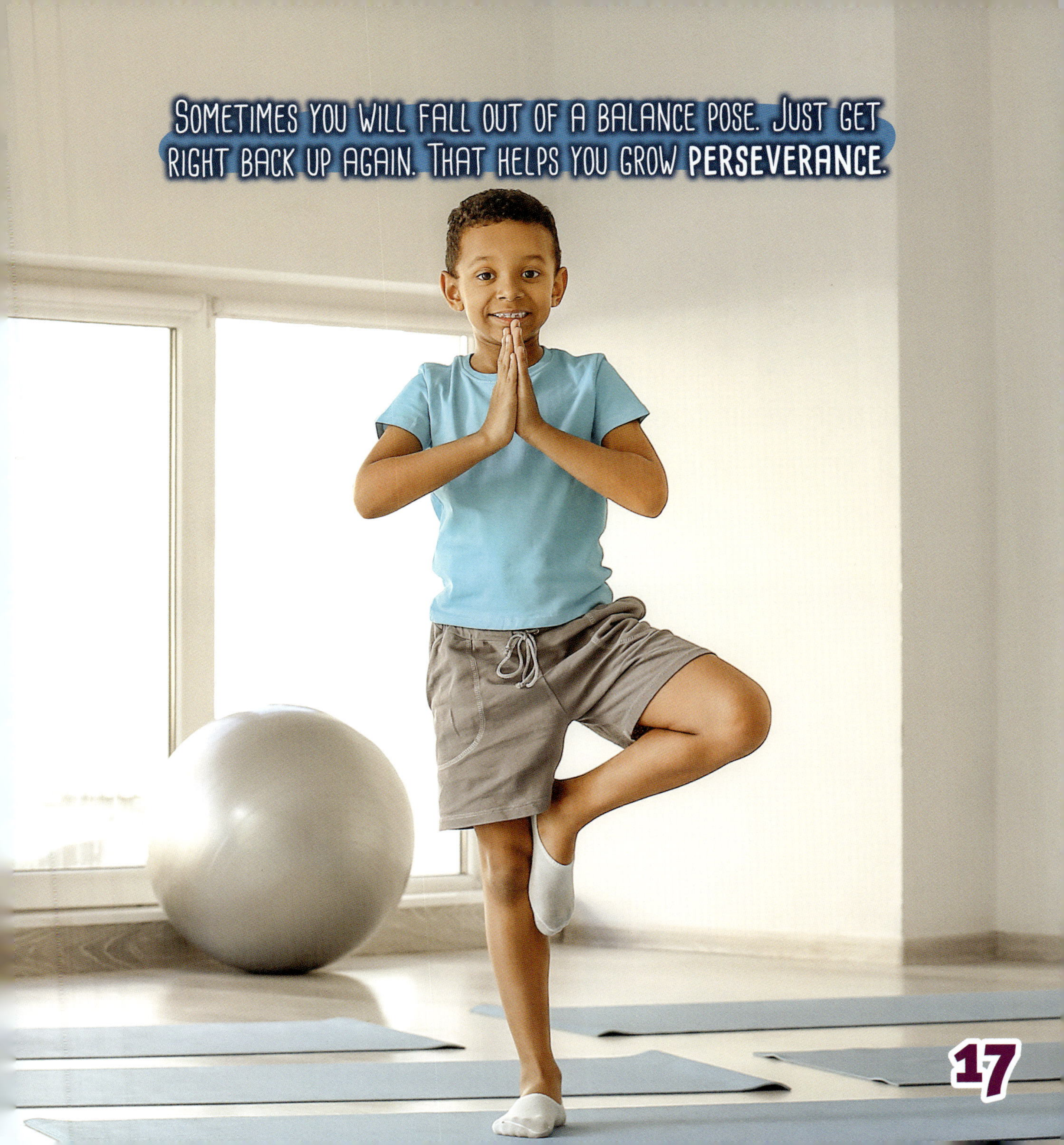

Sometimes you will fall out of a balance pose. Just get right back up again. That helps you grow **perseverance**.

Let It Go

Some poses help you release, or let go, of stress. For seated forward fold, sit up tall with your legs out and arms overhead. Bend forward to touch your toes. It's okay to keep a bend in your knees. You might feel tight in your legs. On your exhales, try to soften your muscles.

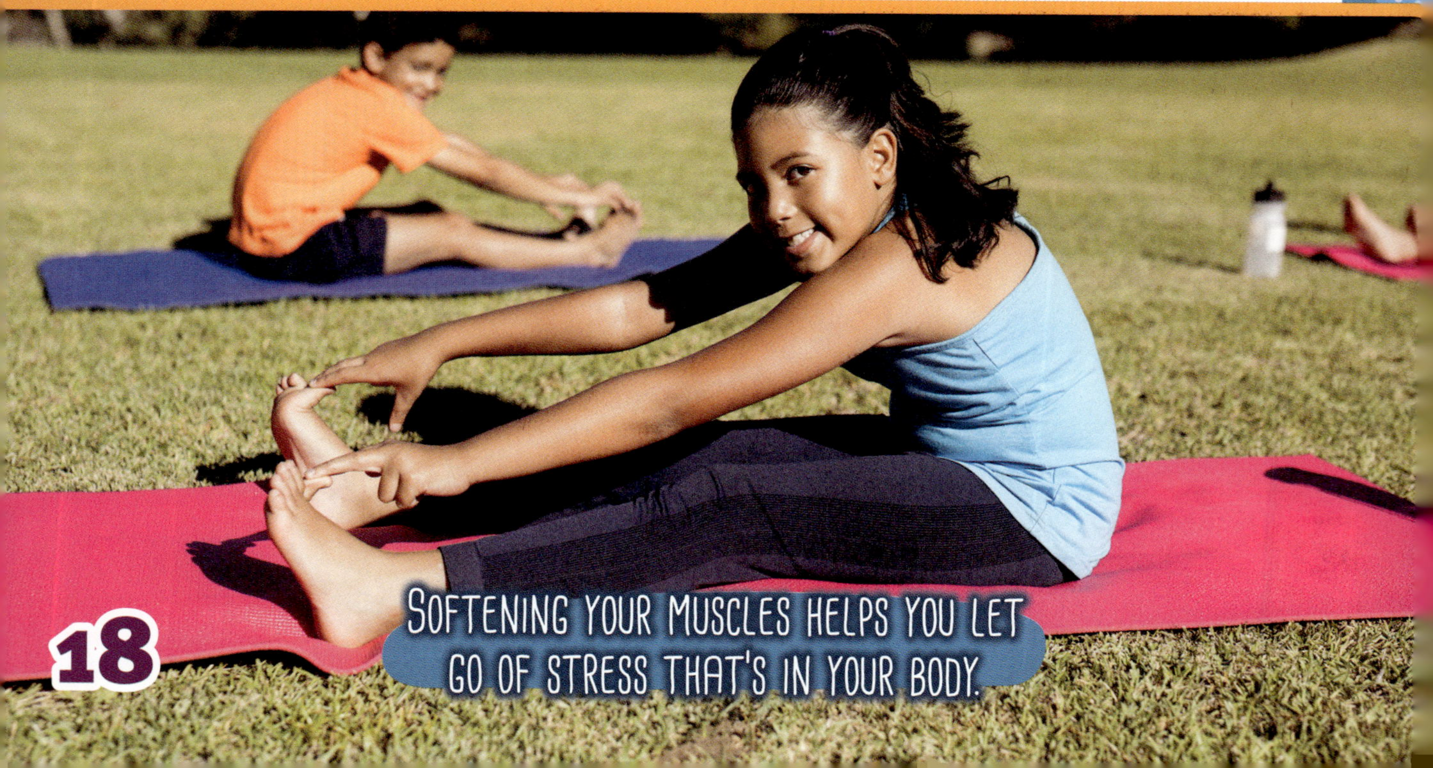

SOFTENING YOUR MUSCLES HELPS YOU LET GO OF STRESS THAT'S IN YOUR BODY.

Many yoga classes end with a pose called *shavasana* (sha-VAH-suh-nuh). It's a relaxation pose. Lay down on your back. Release any tension in your body. Feel your body sink into your mat. Just rest.

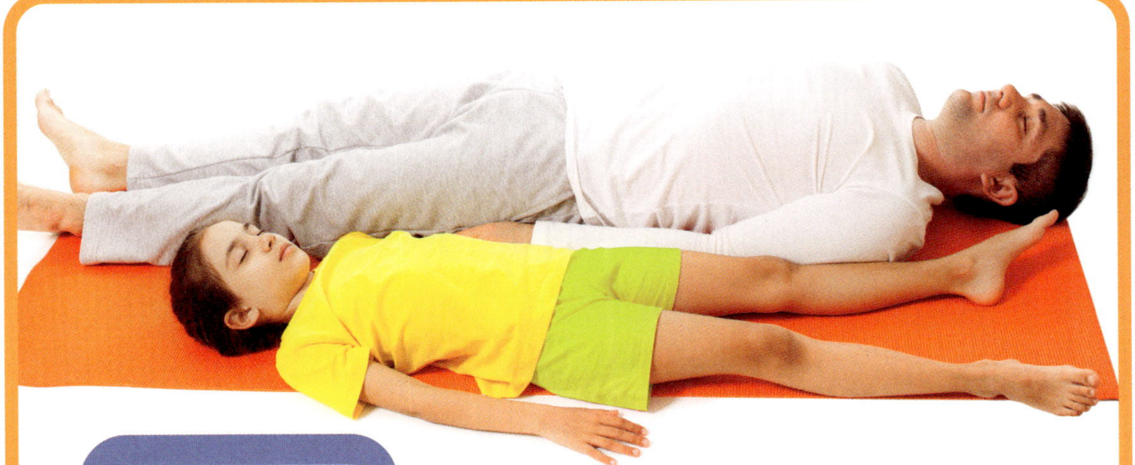

COPING TOOLBOX

IN SHAVASANA, YOU CAN FOCUS ON YOUR BREATH, AS WELL AS YOUR FEELINGS AND THOUGHTS. SEE HOW THEY COME AND GO LIKE A WAVE.

Yoga Every Day

Make sure you follow directions, ask for help, and stay safe while doing yoga. In time, you can create a daily yoga practice. Remember it's more than just good **exercise**. It's a way of life!

When you act with respect and nonviolence, that's yoga. When you focus on your breathing, that's yoga. When you stretch and move with your breath, that's yoga. When you meditate, that's yoga too. Practicing yoga can help you direct your energy, deal with feelings, and find inner peace.

COPING TOOLBOX

YOU CAN PRACTICE YOGA FOR ANY AMOUNT OF TIME. YOU CAN PRACTICE ALONE OR WITH FRIENDS OR A PARENT.

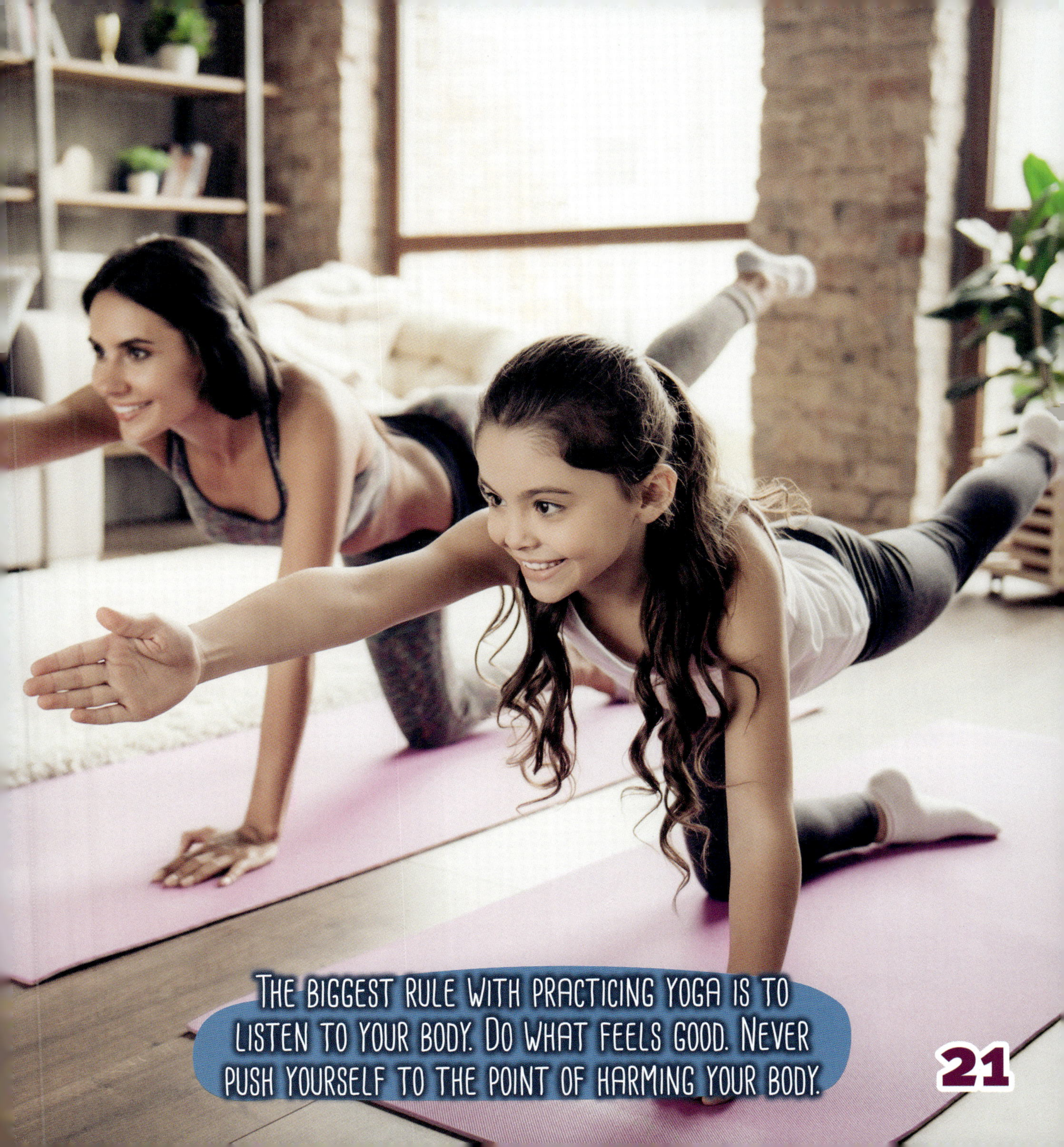

THE BIGGEST RULE WITH PRACTICING YOGA IS TO LISTEN TO YOUR BODY. DO WHAT FEELS GOOD. NEVER PUSH YOURSELF TO THE POINT OF HARMING YOUR BODY.

GLOSSARY

ancient: Having to do with something or someone from long ago.

anxious: Afraid or nervous.

balance: The state in which things occur in equal amounts; the state in which you feel steady.

cope: To deal with and try to find help for problems.

exercise: Activity done to make one's body or mind stronger.

focus: Directed attention.

harmony: Being in agreement or unity.

meditate: To spend time in quiet awareness of one's thoughts.

muscle: A part of the body that makes movement.

nonviolence: Not harming.

perseverance: The quality that allows someone to continue to do something even though it's hard.

pose: A fixed way of holding the body.

Sanskrit: An Indo-European language used in ancient India.

FOR MORE INFORMATION

BOOKS

Anthony, William. *Yoga*. Minneapolis, MN: Bearport Publishing, 2021.

Hoffman, Susannah. *Yoga for Kids*. New York, NY: DK Publishing, 2021.

Stevens, Jamaica. *Yoga Adventure!* Cambridge, MA: Barefoot Books, 2021.

WEBSITES

Kids Yoga Poses
namastekid.com/tool-type/kids-yoga-poses/
Use this library of yoga poses (with pictures) to make your own daily yoga practice!

Peace Out
cosmickids.com/?video_series=peace-out
Listen to guided relaxation meditations with Cosmic Kids.

Yoga for Lowering Stress
kidshealth.org/en/kids/yoga-stress.html
How can yoga help with stress? Find out with KidsHealth.

INDEX